Mediterranean Dinner Cookbook

*Easy and fast recipes to end the day
in the Healthiest way*

Carlo Montesanti

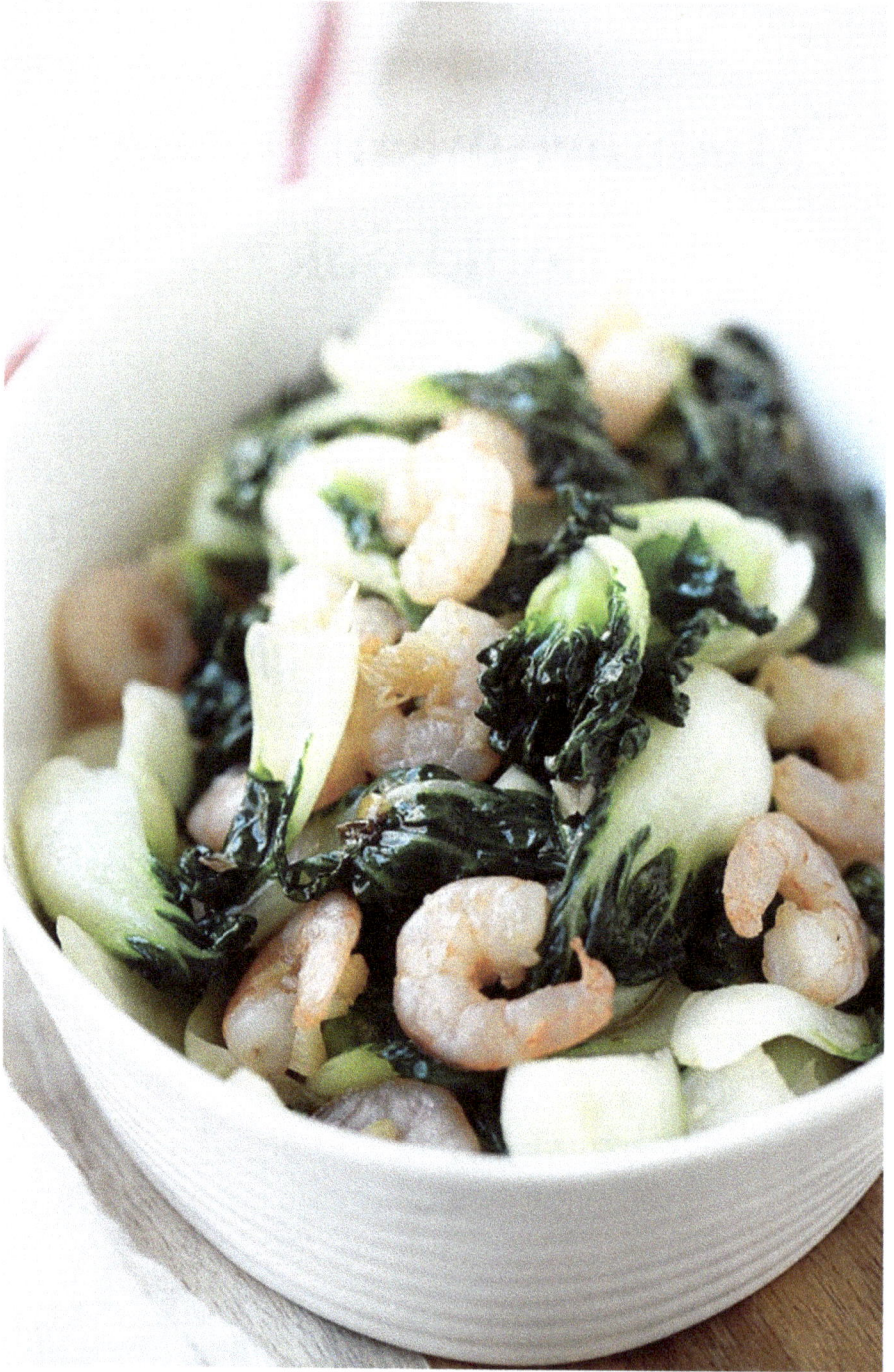

Table of Contents

Prawn & Chili Pak Choi

Prep Time: 30 min

Cook Time: 15 min

Serve: 1

Ingredients:

- 75g (2 ¼ oz.) brown rice

- 1 pak choi

- 60ml (2 fl. oz.) chicken stock

- 1 tbsp. extra virgin olive oil

- 1 garlic clove, finely chopped

- 50g (1 ⅝ oz.) red onion, finely chopped

- ½ bird's eye chili, finely chopped

- 1 tsp freshly grated ginger

- 125g (4 ¼ oz.) shelled raw king prawns

- 1 tbsp. soy sauce

- 1 tsp five-spice

- 1 tbsp. freshly chopped flat-leaf parsley

- A pinch of salt and pepper

Preparation:

1. Bring a medium-sized saucepan of water to the boil and cook the brown rice for 25-30 minutes, or until softened.

2. Tear the pak choi into pieces. Warm the chicken stock in a skillet over medium heat and toss in the pak choi, cooking until the pak choi has slightly wilted.

3. In another skillet, warm olive oil over high heat. Toss in the ginger, chili, red onions and garlic frying for 2-3 minutes. Throw in the prawns, five-spice and soy sauce and cook for 6-8 minutes, or until the cooked throughout. Drain the brown rice and add to the skillet, stirring and cooking for 2-3 minutes. Add the pak choi, garnish with parsley and serve.

Dahl with Kale, Red Onions and Buckwheat

Prep Time: 5 min

Cook Time: 20 min

Serve: 2

Ingredients:

- 1 teaspoon of extra virgin olive oil

- 1 teaspoon of mustard seeds

- 40g (1 ½ oz.) red onions, finely chopped

- 1 clove of garlic, very finely chopped

- 1 teaspoon very finely chopped ginger

- 1 Thai chili, very finely chopped

- 1 teaspoon curry mixture teaspoons turmeric

- 300ml (10 fl. oz.) vegetable broth

- 40g (1 ½ oz.) red lentils

- 50g (1 ⅝ oz.) kale, chopped

- 50ml (1.70 fl. oz.) coconut milk

- 50g (1 ⅝ oz.) buckwheat

Preparation:

1. Heat oil in a pan at medium temperature and add mustard seeds. When they crack, add onion, garlic, ginger and chili. Heat until everything is soft.

2. Add the curry powder and 1 teaspoon of turmeric, mix well. Add the lentils and cook them for 25 to 30 minutes until they are ready.

3. While the lentils are cooking, prepare the buckwheat.

4. Serve buckwheat with the dal.

Chickpeas, Onion, Tomato & Parsley Salad in a Jar

Prep Time: 5 min

Cook Time: 50 min

Serve: 2

Ingredients:

- 1 cup cooked chickpeas

- ½ cup chopped tomatoes

- ½ of a small onion, chopped

- 1 tbsp. chia seeds

- 1 Tbsp. chopped parsley

Dressing:

- 1 tbsp. olive oil and

- 1 tbsp. of Chlorella.

- 1 tbsp. fresh lemon juice and a pinch of sea salt

Preparation:

Put ingredients in this order: dressing, tomatoes, chickpeas, onions and parsley.

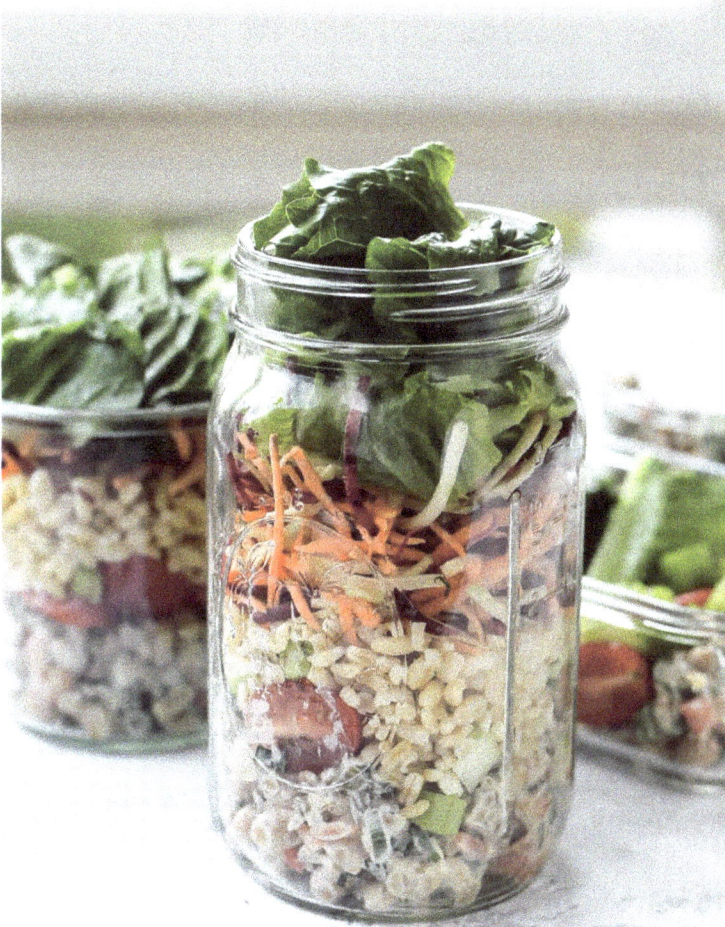

Kale & Feta Salad with Cranberry Dressing

Prep Time: 5 min

Cook Time: 30 min

Serve: 2

Ingredients:

- 9oz kale, finely chopped
- 2oz walnuts, chopped
- 3oz feta cheese, crumbled
- 1 apple, peeled, cored and sliced medjool dates, chopped

For the Dressing:

- 3oz cranberries
- ½ red onion, chopped tablespoons
- olive oil tablespoons water

- teaspoons honey

- 1 tablespoon red wine vinegar

- Sea salt

Preparation:

1. Place the ingredients for the dressing into a food processor and process until smooth. If it seems too thick, you can add a little extra water if necessary. Place all the ingredients for the salad into a bowl.

2. Pour on the dressing and toss the salad until it is well coated in the mixture.

Spiced Fish Tacos with Fresh Corn Salsa

Prep Time: 10 min

Cook Time: 20 min

Serve: 4

Ingredients:

- 1 cup corn

- 1/2 cup red onion, diced

- 1 cup jicama, peeled and chopped

- 1/2 cup red bell pepper, diced

- 1 cup fresh cilantro leaves, finely chopped

- 1 lime, zested and juiced

- tablespoons sour cream tablespoons cayenne pepper

- Salt and pepper to taste

- (4 ounce) fillets tilapia

- tablespoons olive oil corn tortillas, warmed

Preparation:

1. If you do not have any available, you can substitute for water chestnuts, celery, or radishes.

2. Preheat grill for high heat.

For the Corn Salsa:

1. In a medium bowl, mix corn, red onion, jicama, red bell pepper, and cilantro. Stir in lime juice and zest.

2. Brush each fillet with olive oil, and sprinkle with the cayenne and season to taste.

3. Arrange fillets on the grill and cook for 3 minutes per side. For each fish taco, top two corn tortillas with fish, sour cream, and corn salsa.

Sautee Tofu & Kale

Prep Time: 10 min

Cook Time: 10 min

Serve: 3

Ingredients:

- 12 oz. extra firm tofu
- tbsps. olive oil
- ½ tsp. salt & pepper
- 1 tsp. garlic, minced
- 1 bunch kale, chopped

Preparation:

1. Heat oil in a large skillet over medium heat. Fry tofu in a pan for 4-5 minutes. Add kale and stir fry for 3-4 minutes until kale is soft.

2. Add salt, pepper and garlic, and cook for another 1-2 minutes until the garlic is fragrant. Drizzle sesame seeds on top. Serve and enjoy!

Chicken and Lentil Stew

Prep Time: 10 min

Cook Time: 40 min

Serve: 3

Ingredients:

- chicken breasts, diced
- ½ cup red lentils, rinsed
- 1 carrot, chopped
- 1 small onion, chopped
- 1 garlic clove, chopped
- 1 celery stalk, chopped
- 1 small red pepper, chopped
- 1 can tomatoes, chopped
- 1 tbsp. paprika
- 1 tsp ginger, grated

- tbsp. extra virgin olive oil

- ½ cup fresh parsley leaves, finely cut, to serve

Preparation:

1. Heat olive oil in a casserole and gently brown the chicken, stirring. Add in onions, garlic, celery, carrot, pepper, paprika and ginger.

2. Cook, constantly stirring, for 2-3 minutes. Add in the lentils and tomatoes and bring to a boil.

3. Lower heat, cover, and simmer for 30 minutes, or until the lentils are tender and the chicken is cooked through.

4. Serve sprinkled with fresh parsley.

Mussels in Red Wine Sauce

Prep Time: 10 min

Cook Time: 25 min

Serve: 2

Ingredients:

- 800g (2lb) mussels

- x 400g (14oz) tins of chopped tomatoes

- 25g (1oz) butter

- 1 tablespoon fresh chives, chopped

- 1 tablespoon fresh parsley, chopped

- 1 bird's-eye chilli, finely chopped

- cloves of garlic, crushed

- 400mls (14fl oz.) red wine

- Juice of 1 lemon

Preparation:

1. Wash the mussels, remove their beards and set them aside. Heat the butter in a large saucepan and add in the red wine. Reduce the heat and add the parsley, chives, chilli and garlic while stirring.

2. Add in the tomatoes, lemon juice and mussels. Cover the saucepan and cook for 2-3. Remove the saucepan from the heat and take out any mussels which haven't opened and discard them. Serve and eat immediately.

Breakfast Salad from Grains and Fruits

Prep Time: 15 min

Cook Time: 20 min

Serve: 6

Ingredients:

- ¼ tsp. salt

- ¾ cup bulgur

- ¾ cup quick cooking brown rice

- 1 8-oz. low fat vanilla yogurt

- 1 cup raisins

- 1 Granny Smith apple

- 1 orange

- 1 Red delicious apple

- 3 cups water

Preparation:

1. On high fire, place a large pot and bring water to a boil. Add bulgur and rice. Lower fire to a simmer and cook for ten minutes while covered. Turn off fire, set aside for 2 minutes while covered. In baking sheet, transfer and evenly spread grains to cool.

2. Meanwhile, peel oranges and cut into sections. Chop and core apples. Once grains are cool, transfer to a large serving bowl along with fruits. Add yogurt and mix well to coat. Serve and enjoy.

Delicious Rice and Spinach

Prep Time: 10 min

Cook Time: 15 min

Serve: 6

Ingredients:

- 1 onion

- 2 pinch sea salt

- 2 pinch black pepper.

- 1 cup unsalted vegetable broth

- 2 tablespoons olive oil.

- 2 can brown rice

- 4 cups fresh baby spinach

- Juice of orange

- 1 garlic clove

- 1 orange Zest

Preparation:

1. In a substantial skillet over medium-high heat the olive oil until it gleams. Include the onion and for around 5 minutes blending infrequently until delicate.

2. Include the spinach and **for** around 2 minutes blending infrequently until it fades. Include the garlic and for 30 seconds blending continually. Blend in the orange juice soup ocean salt and pepper. Convey to a stew.

3. Mix in the rice and for around 4 minutes mixing until the rice is warmed through and the fluid is consumed.

Blue Cheese and Grains Salad

Prep Time: 15 min

Cook Time: 40 min

Serve: 4

Ingredients:

- ¼ cup thinly sliced scallions

- ½ cup millet, rinsed

- ½ cup quinoa, rinsed

- 1 ½ tsp. olive oil

- 1 garlic, minced

- Oz. blue cheese

- 2 tbsp. fresh lemon juice

- 2 tsp. dried rosemary

- 4-oz. boneless, skinless chicken breasts

- 6 oz. baby spinach

- olive oil

- cooking spray

Dressing:

- ¼ cup fresh raspberries

- 1 tbsp. pure maple syrup

- 1 tsp. fresh thyme leaf

- 2 tbsp. grainy mustard

- 6 tbsp. balsamic vinegar

Preparation:

1. Bring millet, quinoa, and 2 ¼ cups water on a small saucepan to a boil. Once boiling, slow fire to a simmer and stir. Cover and cook until water is fully absorbed and grains are soft around 15 minutes.

2. Turn off fire, fluff grains with a fork and set aside to cool a bit. Arrange one oven rack to highest position and preheat broiler. Line a baking sheet with foil, and grease

with cooking spray. Whisk well pepper, oil, rosemary, lemon juice and garlic.

3. Rub onto chicken. Place chicken on prepared pan, pop into the broiler and broil until juices run clear and no longer pin inside around 12 minutes. Meanwhile, make the dressing by combining all ingredients in a blender. Blend until smooth. Remove chicken from oven, cool slightly before cutting into strips, against the grain.

4. To assemble, place grains in a large salad bowl. Add in dressing and spinach, toss to mix well.

Add scallions and pear, mix gently and evenly divide into four plates. Top each salad with cheese and chicken.

5. Serve and enjoy.

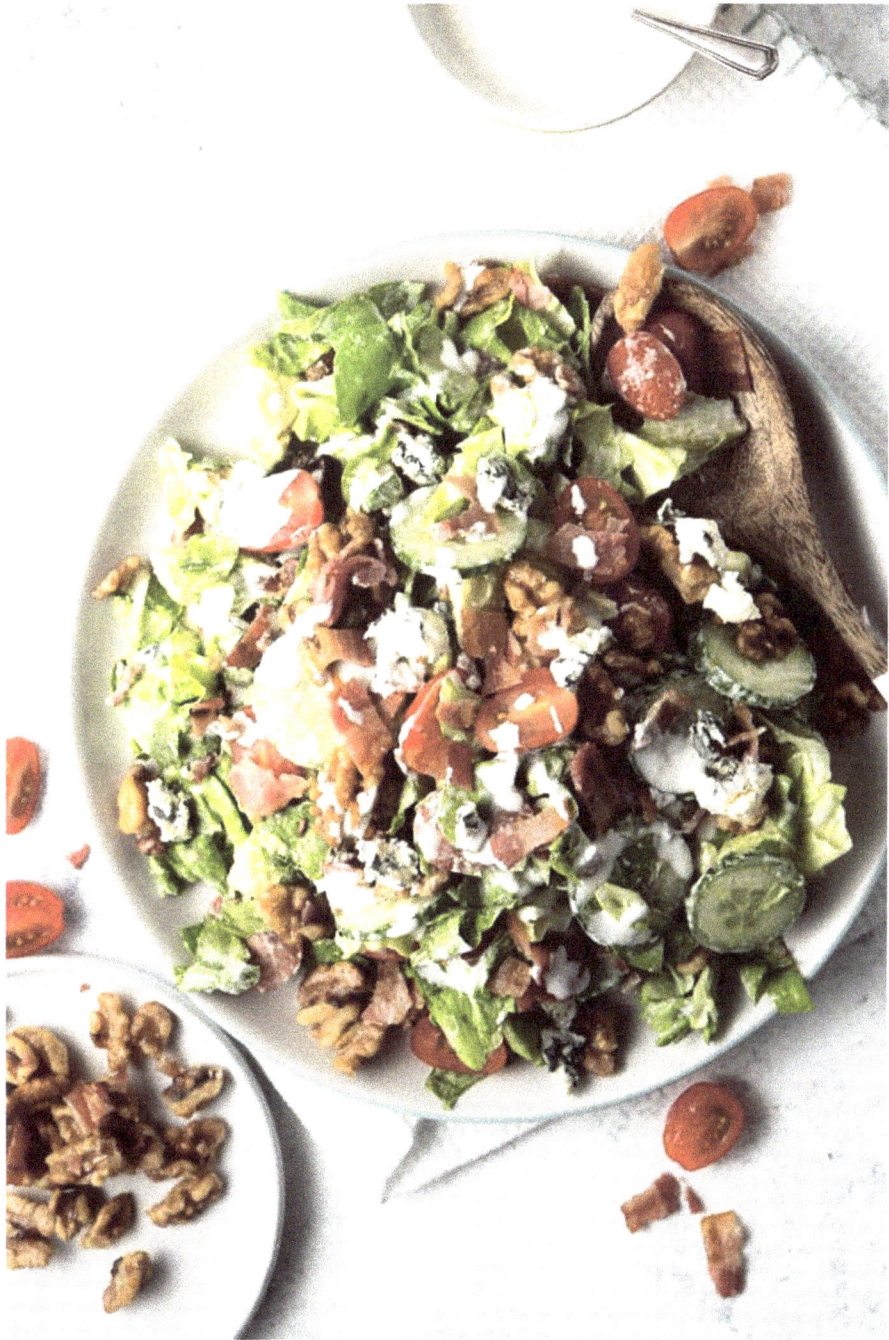

Cucumber Salad with Rice and Asparagus

Prep Time: 15 min

Cook Time: 21 min

Serve: 6

Ingredients:

- 4 heads butter lettuce

- ¼ cup chopped fresh dill

- 2 ½ tbsp. Vegetable oil

- ½ tsp. dry mustard

- 1 tbsp. white wine vinegar

- 1 tbsp. white sugar

- 2 tbsp. Dijon mustard

- 3 green onions, chopped

- 1 ½ cups English cucumber, peeled, seeded and chopped
- 1 lb. thin asparagus spears, trimmed and cut into 1-inch
- 1 cup long grain white rice
- 1 ¾ cups water

Preparation:

1. Bring to a boil 1 ¾ cups water in a medium saucepan. Add rice and bring again to a boil. Once boiling, reduce fire to low. Continue cooking around 20 minutes or until water is fully absorbed and rice is tender. Turn of fire and fluff rice with a fork and transfer to a bowl to cool.

2. For 1 minute, cook asparagus in boiling and salted water. Drain and rinse asparagus and cut into 1-inch long pieces.

3. Mix rice, green onions, cucumber and asparagus thoroughly. Cover and chill. In a separate medium bowl, stir thoroughly chopped dill, oil, dry mustard, vinegar,

sugar and mustard. Cover and chill. Mix dressing and salad and season with pepper and salt to taste.

4. Then, in a large bowl lined with lettuce, transfer the rice salad and garnish with dill sprigs. Serve and enjoy.

Mexican Baked Beans and Rice

Prep Time: 30 min

Cook Time: 45 min

Serve: 6

Ingredients:

- 1 ½ cups cooked brown rice

- 1 15-oz. can no-salt added black beans, drained and rinsed

- 1 cup chopped poblano pepper

- 1 cup chopped red bell pepper

- 1 cup frozen yellow corn

- 1 cup shredded reduced fat Monterey Jack cheese

- 1 lb. skinless, boneless chicken breast cut into bite sized pieces

- 1 tbsp. chili powder

- 1 tbsp. cumin

- 2 14.5-oz. cans no salt added tomatoes, diced or crushed

- 4 garlic cloves, crushed

Preparation:

1. With cooking spray, grease a 3-quart shallow casserole and preheat oven to 4000F. Spread cooked brown rice in bottom of casserole. Layer chicken on top of brown rice.

2. Mix well garlic, seasonings, peppers, corn, beans and tomatoes in a medium bowl. Evenly spread bean mixture on top of chicken. Sprinkle cheese on top of beans and pop into the oven. Bake for 45 minutes, remove from oven and serve.

Raisins, Nuts and Beef on Hashweh Rice

Prep Time: 20 min

Cook Time: 50 min

Serve: 8

Ingredients:

- ½ cup dark raisins, soaked in

- 2 cups water for an hour

- 1/3 cup slivered almonds, toasted and soaked in

- 2 cups water overnight

- 1/3 cup pine nuts, toasted and soaked in

- 2 cups water overnight

- ½ cup fresh parsley leaves, roughly chopped

- pepper and salt to taste

- ¾ tsp. ground cinnamon, divided

- ¾ tsp. cloves, divided

- 1 tsp. garlic powder

- 1 ¾ tsp. allspice, divided

- 1 lb. lean ground beef or lean ground lamb

- 1 small red onion, finely chopped

- Olive oil

- 1 ½ cups medium grain rice

Preparation:

1. For 15 to 20 minutes, soak rice in cold water. You will know that soaking is enough when you can snap a grain of rice easily between your thumb and index finger. Once soaking is done, drain rice well.

2. Meanwhile, drain pine nuts, almonds and raisins for at least a minute and transfer to one bowl. Set aside. On a heavy cooking pot on medium high fire, heat 1 tbsp. olive oil. Once oil is hot, add red onions. Sauté for a minute before adding ground meat and sauté for another minute.

3. Season ground meat with pepper, salt, ½ tsp. ground cinnamon, ½ tsp. ground cloves, 1 tsp. garlic powder, and 1 ¼ tsp. allspice. Sauté ground meat for 10 minutes or until browned and cooked fully. Drain fat.

4. In same pot with cooked ground meat, add rice on top of meat. Season with a bit of pepper and salt. Add remaining cinnamon, ground cloves, and allspice. Do not mix.

5. Add 1 tbsp. olive oil and 2 ½ cups of water. Bring to a boil and once boiling, lower fire to a simmer. Cook while covered until liquid is fully absorbed, around 20 to 25 minutes. Turn of fire.

6. To serve, place a large serving platter that fully covers the mouth of the pot. Place platter upside down on mouth of pot, and invert pot. The pot's inside should now rest on the platter with the rice on the bottom of the plate and ground meat on top of it. Garnish the top of the meat with raisins, almonds, pine nuts, and parsley. Serve and enjoy.

Fried Rice

Prep Time: 10 min

Cook Time: 20 min

Serve: 4

Ingredients:

- 4 cups cold cooked rice

- 1/2 cup peas

- 1 medium yellow onion, diced

- 5 tbsp. olive oil

- 4 oz. frozen medium shrimp, thawed, shelled, deveined and chopped finely

- 6 oz. roast pork

- 3 large eggs

- Salt and freshly ground black pepper

- 1/2 tsp. cornstarch

Preparation:

1. Combine the salt and ground black pepper and 1/2 tsp. cornstarch, coat the shrimp with it. Chop the roasted pork. Beat the eggs and set aside.

2. Stir-fry the shrimp in a wok on high fire with 1 tbsp. heated oil until pink, around 3 minutes. Set the shrimp aside and stir fry the roasted pork briefly. Remove both from the pan.

3. In the same pan, stir-fry the onion until soft, Stir the peas and cook until bright green. Remove both from pan. Add 2 tbsp. oil in the same pan, add the cooked rice. Stir and separate the individual grains. Add the beaten eggs, toss the rice. Add the roasted pork, shrimp, vegetables and onion.

4. Toss everything together. Season with salt and pepper to taste.

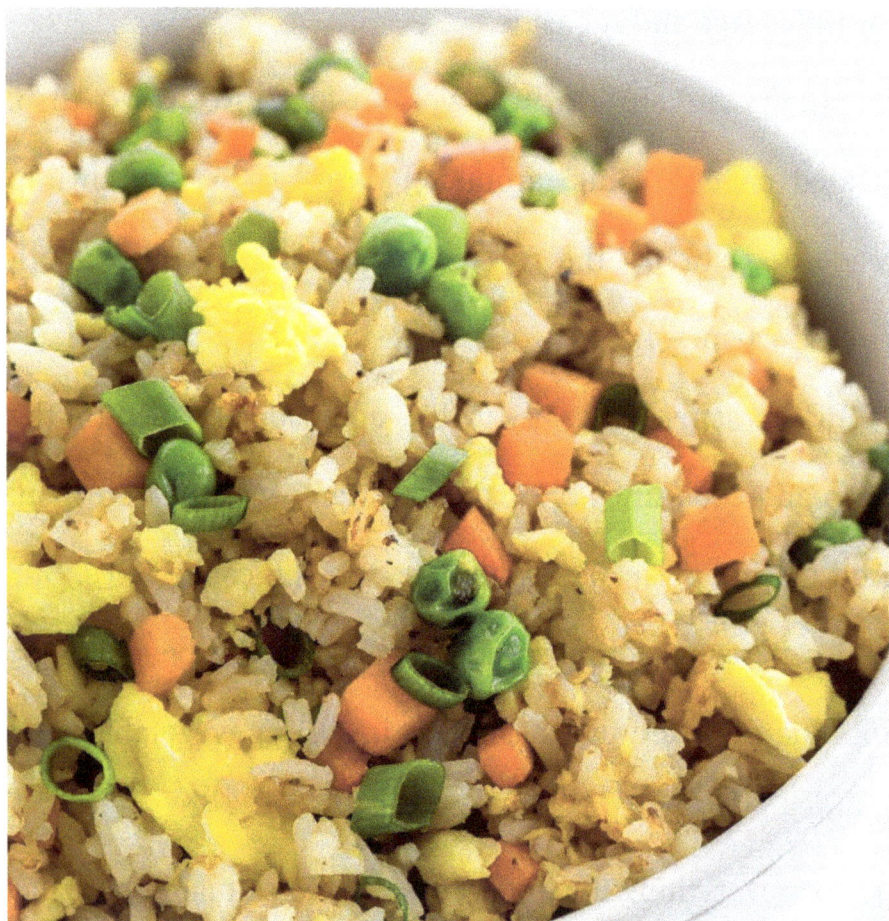

Rice & Currant Salad

Mediterranean Style

Prep Time: 30 min

Cook Time: 50 min

Serve: 4

Ingredients:

- 1 cup basmati rice salt

- 2 1/2 Tablespoons lemon juice

- 1 teaspoon grated orange zest

- 2 Tablespoons fresh orange juice

- 1/4 cup olive oil

- 1/2 teaspoon cinnamon

- Salt and pepper to taste

- 4 chopped green onions

- 1/2 cup dried currants

- 3/4 cup shelled pistachios or almonds

- 1/4 cup chopped fresh parsley

Preparation:

1. Place a nonstick pot on medium high fire and add rice. Toast rice until opaque and starts to smell, around 10 minutes. Add 4 quarts of boiling water to pot and 2 tsp. salt. 2. Boil until tender, around 8 minutes uncovered. Drain the rice and spread out on a lined cookie sheet to cool completely. In a large salad bowl, whisk well the oil, juices and spices. Add salt and pepper to taste.

3. Add half of the green onions, half of parsley, currants, and nuts. Toss with the cooled rice and let stand for at least 20 minutes. If needed adjust seasoning with pepper and salt. Garnish with remaining parsley and green onions.

Carrot and Bran Mini Muffins

Prep Time: 10 min

Cook Time: 18 min

Serve: 18

Ingredients:

- Nonstick cooking spray

- 1 cup oat bran

- 1 cup whole-wheat flour

- ½ cup all-purpose flour

- ½ cup old-fashioned oats

- 3 tablespoons packed brown sugar

- 1 teaspoon baking soda

- 1 teaspoon baking powder

- 2 teaspoons ground cinnamon

- 2 teaspoons ground ginger

- ½ teaspoon ground nutmeg

- ¼ teaspoon sea salt

- 1¼ cups unsweetened almond milk

- 2 tablespoons honey

- 1 egg

- 2 tablespoons extra-virgin olive oil

- 1½ cups grated carrots

- ¼ cup raisins

Preparation:

1. Preheat the oven to 350°F. Line two mini muffin tins with paper liners, or coat with nonstick cooking spray.

2. In a large bowl, whisk the oat bran, whole-wheat and all-purpose flours, oats, brown sugar, baking soda, baking powder, cinnamon, ginger, nutmeg, and salt. Set aside.

3. In a medium bowl, whisk the almond milk, honey, egg, and olive oil. Add the wet ingredients to the dry ingredients

and fold until just blended. The batter will be lumpy with streaks of flour remaining. Fold in the carrots and raisins.

4. Fill each muffin cup three-fourths full. Bake for 15 to 18 minutes, until a toothpick inserted in the center of a muffin comes out clean. Cool on a wire rack before serving.

French Toast

Prep Time: 20 min

Cook Time: 10 min

Serve: 6

Ingredients:

- 1½ cups unsweetened almond milk

- 2 eggs, beaten

- 2 egg whites, beaten

- 1 teaspoon vanilla extract

- Zest of 1 orange

- Juice of 1 orange

- 1 teaspoon ground nutmeg

- 6 light whole-wheat bread slices

- Nonstick cooking spray

Preparation:

1. In a small bowl, whisk the almond milk, eggs, egg whites, vanilla, orange zest and juice, and nutmeg.

2. Arrange the bread in a single layer in a 9-by-13-inch baking dish. Pour the milk and egg mixture over the top. Allow the bread to soak for about 10 minutes, turning once.

3. Spray a nonstick skillet with cooking spray and heat over medium-high heat. Working in batches, add the bread and cook for about 5 minutes per side until the custard sets.

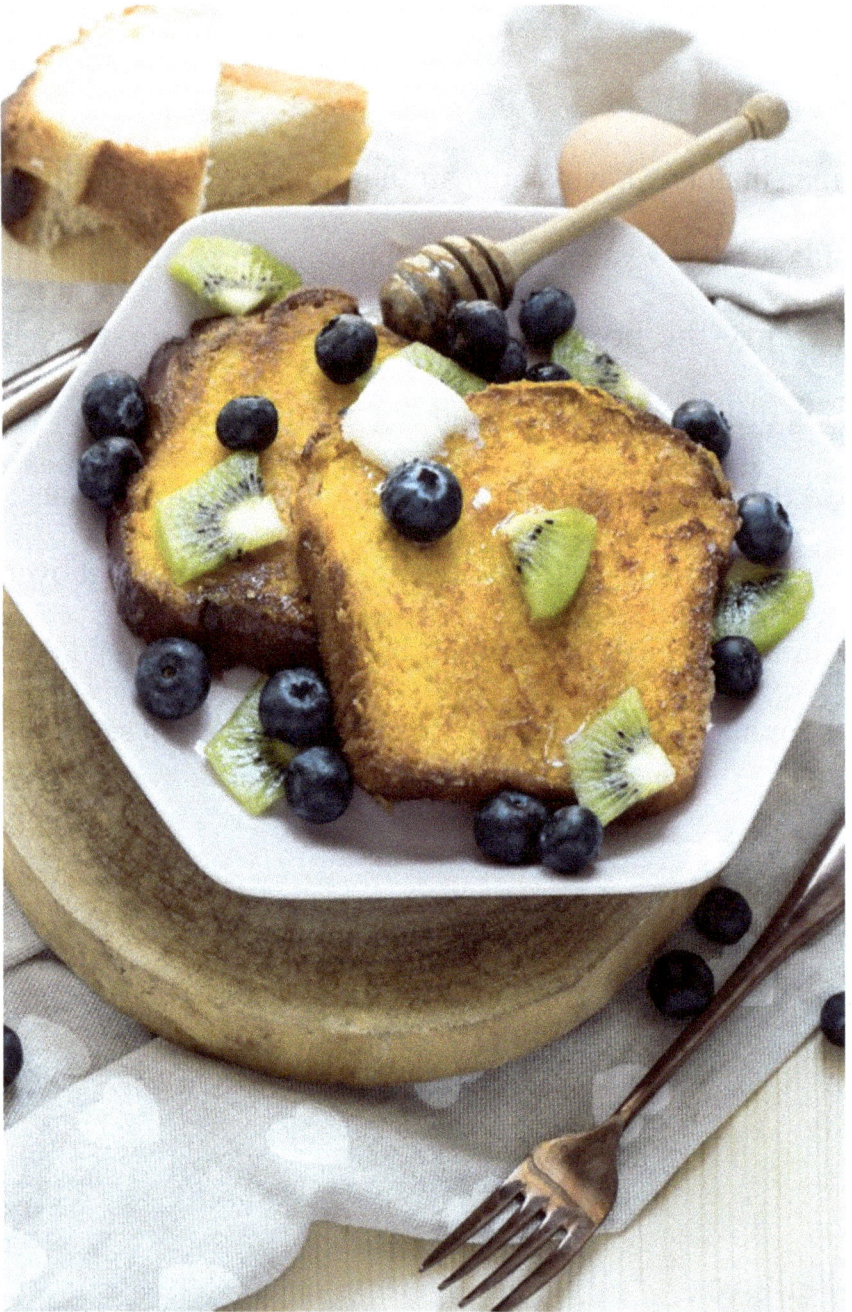

Tomato and Zucchini Frittata

Prep Time: 10 min

Cook Time: 18 min

Serve: 4

Ingredients:

- 3 eggs

- 3 egg whites

- ½ cup unsweetened almond milk

- ½ teaspoon sea salt

- ⅛ Teaspoon freshly ground black pepper

- 2 tablespoons extra-virgin olive oil

- 1 zucchini, chopped

- 8 cherry tomatoes, halved

- ¼ cup (about 2 ounces) grated Parmesan cheese

Preparation:

1. Heat the oven's broiler to high, adjusting the oven rack to the center position. In a small bowl, whisk the eggs, egg whites, almond milk, sea salt, and pepper. Set aside.

2. In a 12-inch ovenproof skillet over medium-high heat, heat the olive oil until it shimmers. Add the zucchini and tomatoes and cook for 5 minutes, stirring occasionally. Pour the egg mixture over the vegetables and cook for about 4 minutes without stirring until the eggs set around the edges.

3. Using a silicone spatula, pull the set eggs away from the edges of the pan. Tilt the pan in all directions to allow the unset eggs to fill the spaces along the edges. Continue to cook for about 4 minutes more without stirring until the edges set again.

4. Sprinkle the eggs with the Parmesan. Transfer the pan to the broiler. Cook for 3 to 5 minutes until the cheese melts and the eggs are puffy. Cut into wedges to serve.

Mediterranean Pork Chops

Total Time: 30 min

Serve: 2

Ingredients:

- Bone-in pork chops (or boneless pork chops) - 2

- Olive oil - 1 tablespoon

- Ragu chunky pasta sauce (1 lb. 8 oz.) - ½ jar

- Red or green bell pepper (large, sliced) - ½

Preparation:

1. Cook pork chops inside 1 of tablespoon olive oil set at medium to high heat in a 12-inch pan. Cook until pork chop appears brown and remove from the pan. Cook green pepper until it is tender using the remaining 1 tablespoon olive oil using the same pan as before, and until tender.

2. Add Pasta Sauce to the pan and set to high heat Mix properly until the mixture starts to boil. Set heat to low and put pork chops back into the pan.

3. Close the lid and leave to simmer for about 10 minutes or until pork is thoroughly cooked.

Pesto chicken pasta

Prep Time: 5 min

Cook Time: 20 min

Serve: 3

Ingredients:

- Two garlic cloves

- 1/2 lb penne pasta

- 1 cup milk

- 1 lb boneless chicken breast

- 2 tbsp butter

- 3 oz cream cheese

- 1/3 cup basil pesto

- 1/4 cup grated Parmesan

- 1.5 cups chicken broth

- Black pepper

- One pinch of red pepper

Preparation:

1. Take the chicken breast piece & cut them into 1-inch pieces. Then add butter to a frypan & melt it.

2. Cook chicken until it turns to brown over medium heat.

3. Add the chopped garlic to it. Add garlic and chicken to the frying pan and cook it for one minute.

4. Add pasta & chicken broth to the garlic and chicken mixture. Put a lid on the frypan, boil the broth on high flame. After the broth is fully boiled, mix paste and heat on low flame for eight minutes. Once the pasta is tender & most broth is soaked up, add cream cheese, milk, and pesto.

5. Stir it & cook over high temp till the cream cheese melts fully. Lastly, add the chopped parmesan and mix it until fully combined. If using, add the spinach & sliced sun-dried tomatoes. Mix until the spinach has wilted, remove pasta

from the stove. Decorate pasta with crushed pepper & a pinch of red pepper & serve.

Spinach pesto pasta

Prep Time: 10 min

Cook Time: 15 min

Serve: 4

Ingredients:

- 1/2 cup peas

- One whole ripe avocado

- 2 cups baby spinach leaves

- 7 tbsp basil pesto

- 12 oz of fusilli pasta

- Salt to taste

- 1.5 tbsp red wine vinegar

- 1/2 tsp black pepper

Preparation:

Cook pasta in boiling water for ten minutes. Transfer the hot pasta over spinach in a bowl. Add pasta liquid to the bowl. Mix vinegar, pepper, peas, pepper, and avocado. Serve and enjoy it.

Fiber packed chicken rice

Prep Time: 5 min

Cook Time: 10 min

Serve: 2

Ingredients:

- 1 tsp rice vinegar

- 1 tsp toasted sesame oil

- Six scallions root

- One shredded carrot

- 1 tbsp avocado oil

- Three eggs

- One pinch of salt

- Black pepper

- 1/2 cup peas

- 2 cups cooked brown rice

- 3 tsp soy sauce

- 1/2 tsp grated ginger

Preparation:

1. Take ½ tbsp of olive oil & heat it. Take eggs in a bowl & whisk until well combined & put a pinch of salt & black pepper powder. Pour these eggs into a saucepan & scramble.

2. Now add half tbsp olive oil in a pan & add scallion & carrots. Sauté the ingredients till they are softened (3-4 min). Take frozen peas in a pan & add rice, vinegar, tamari, ginger & sesame oil. Mix them well. Now turn off the heat & combine with scrambled eggs.

3. Now add salt according to taste. Now cook the whole dish for almost 5-5 min until it is well cooked and warmed.

4. Bean sprouts, veggie & water chestnuts will be a delicious addition to the dish if needed.

Oven-Poached Salmon Fillets

Prep Time: 5 min

Cook Time: 30 min

Serve: 4

Ingredients:

- 1 tbsp pepper

- 2 tbsp dry white wine

- 1 lb salmon fillet

- 1 Lemon wedges, for garnish

- 1 2 tbsp chopped shallot

- ¼ tsp salt

Preparation:

1. Whisk all the items except salmon in a bowl. Put salmon in baking tray sprayed with oil with skin placed downwards.

2. Pour the bowl content over the salmon and bake for 25 minutes in a preheated oven at 425 degrees.

3. Serve with wedges.

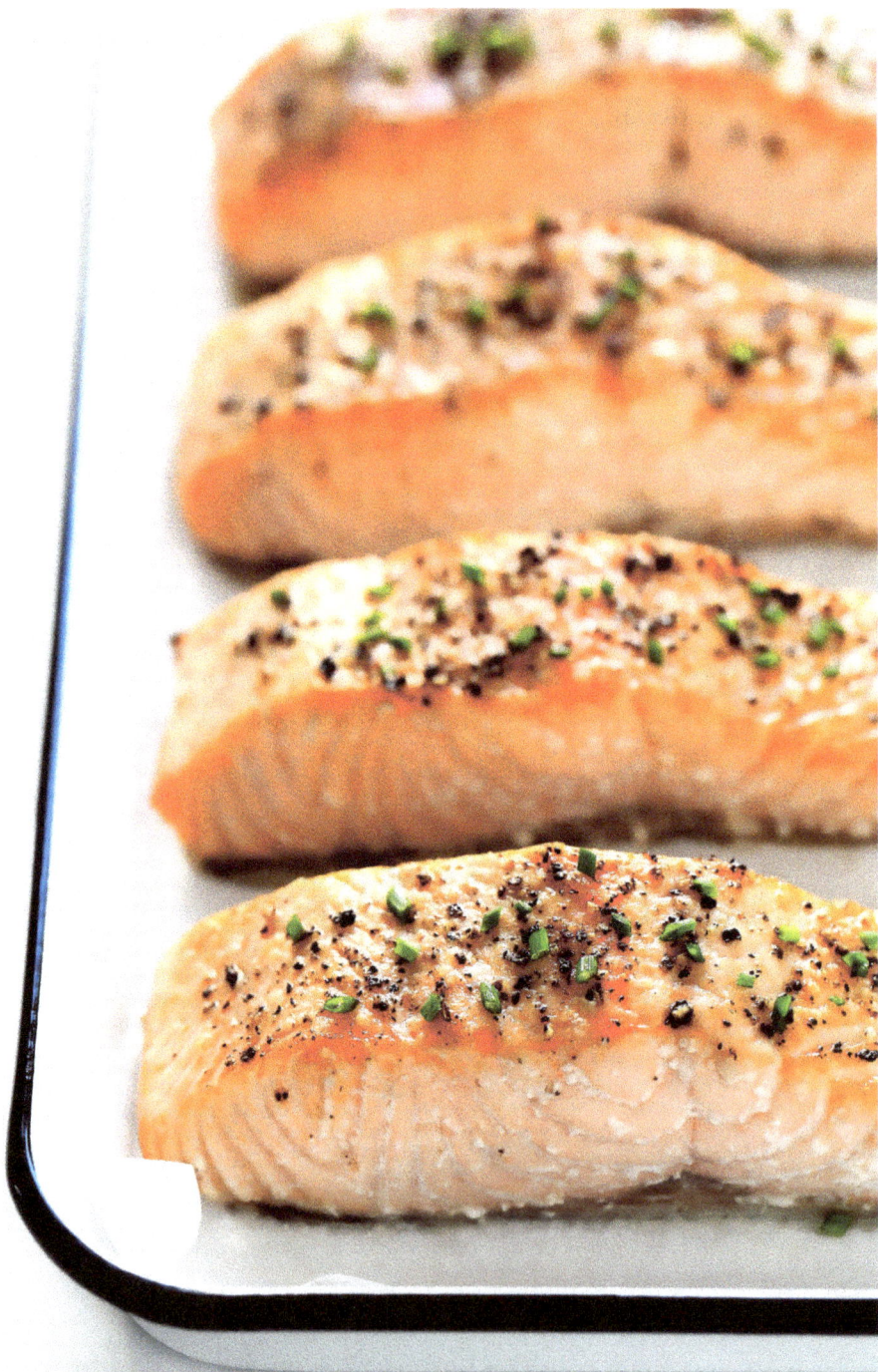

Herb rice

Prep Time: 5 min

Cook Time: 20 min

Serve: 4

Ingredients:

- 1 tsp salt

- 2 Tbsp butter

- 1 tsp onion black pepper juice

- 3 cup chicken broth

- 1 tsp garlic

- 1/4 cup lemon juice

- 1.5 cup basmati rice

- 1/2 tsp rosemary, basil, dill, parsley, oregano, thyme

Preparation:

1. Melt butter on moderate heat & add salt & black pepper powder. Keep stirring till the onion is softened. Now add garlic & cook (1 min).

2. Add chicken broth & lemon juice with herb along with rice. Keep stirring until mixed. Now, wait for a boil, cover & lower heat. Keep cooking until rice is well softened & garnish with herbs if required. Serve & enjoy.

Easy Apricot Biscotti

Prep Time: 20 min

Cook Time: 50 min

Serve: 24

Ingredients:

- 2 Tablespoon Olive Oil

- ¼ Cup Almonds, Chopped Course

- ¾ Cup Whole Wheat Flour

- ½ Teaspoon Almond Extract, Pure

- 2/3 Cup Dried Apricots, Chopped

- 2 Tablespoons Dark Honey, Raw

- 2 Eggs, Lightly Beaten

- 1 Teaspoon Baking Powder

- ¼ Cup Brown Sugar

- 2 Tablespoons Milk, 1%

- ¾ Cup All Purpose Flour

Preparation:

1. Preheat your stove to 350, and then get out a bowl. Whisk your all-purpose whole wheat flour and baking powder together. Add in your milk, honey, canola oil, eggs and almond extract together. Stir until it become a dough like consistency and then add in your almonds and apricots.

2. Place flours on your hands and then mix everything. Place your dough on a cookie sheet and flatten it to be about a foot long and three inches wide. It should be about an inch tall.

3. Bake for twenty-five to thirty minutes. It should be light brown. Take it out and allow it to cool for ten to fifteen minutes. Cut into twenty- four slices by cutting crosswise.

4. Arrange the cut slices face down on the baking sheet, baking for another fifteen to twenty minutes. It should be crisp, and allow it to cool before serving.

Garden salad with orange and olive

Prep Time: 15 min

Cook Time: 0 min

Serve: 4

Ingredients:

- Five oranges

- 4 cups rocket spinach

- 150 g feta

- 1 cup olives

- 2 tbsp olive oil

- A pinch of salt

- One clove garlic

Preparation:

1. Peel & dice 4 of the oranges Combine oranges, olives & leaves in a bowl. Crumble feta over the top of the salad.

2. Whisk together the final orange juice, olive oil, salt, and as much garlic as you like. Taste & adjust seasoning according to requirement.

3. Pour dressing on the salad & toss gently to mix well.

Chickpea Sunflower Sandwich

Prep Time: 20 min

Cook Time: 0 min

Serve: 4

Ingredients:

- Garlic Herb Sauce

- 1 tbsp Lemon juice

- ¼ cup Prepared hummus

- 2 tbsp dill

- Water as needed

- Two minced Garlic cloves

- Chickpea Sunflower Sandwich

- 1 tbsp Maple syrup

- ¼ cup Sunflower seeds roasted

- 15 oz chickpeas

- 3 tbsp Mayonnaise

- 1/2 tsp Dijon or spicy mustard

- Pepper to taste

- ¼ chopped Red onion

- Eight slices of wheat bread

- 2 tbsp dill

- Optional Toppings

- Lettuce

- Sliced avocado Tomato

- Onion

Preparation:

1. To prepare the sauce (garlic herb): mix minced garlic, dill, lemon, and hummus in a bowl. Now set aside.

2. In another bowl, mash the chickpeas roughly. To add texture, leave some in large chunks. Then add vegan mayo or tahini, sunflower seeds, maple syrup, mustard, chopped dill, pepper, and red onion. Mix them.

3. Toast bread in vegan oil or butter (optional).

4. Take four slices of bread. Scoop your sunflower seed filling and chickpeas on them. Add the garlic herb sauce along with your optional toppings. Top with the more four slices of bread to form a sandwich.

Balsamic Vinaigrette

Prep Time: 4 min

Cook Time: 0 min

Serve: 4

Ingredients:

- ¼ cup Balsamic vinegar

- 1 tbsp Dijon mustard

- 2 tbsp Honey

- ¾ cup Canola Oil

- One Garlic clove

- ½ tsp black pepper

- 1 tsp Poppyseed

Preparation:

Take a food processor and blend all ingredients in it for 3-4 minutes, thoroughly emulsified. (You can also take a jar and shake all the ingredients vigorously in it, as an alternative)

Easy Chia Seed Pudding

Prep Time: 5 min

Cook Time: 0 min

Serve: 4

Ingredients:

- ½ cup Chia Seeds

- 1.5 cup of rice milk

- 1 tsp Vanilla Extract

- ¼ tsp Cinnamon

- ¼ cup Maple Syrup

Preparation:

1. Take a bowl or a mason jar, add the chia seeds, maple syrup, vanilla, rice milk, and cinnamon. Mix well!

2. Make sure chia seeds do not stick to container sides. Cover the mixture and refrigerate (at least 4 hours or even overnight). You can also add fruit (optional) before serving.

Herb Pesto

Prep Time: 5 min

Cook Time: 0 min

Serve: 4-5

Ingredients:

- ½ cup Parsley leaves
- 1 cup basil leaves
- 2 Garlic cloves
- ½ cup Oregano leaves
- 2 tbsp lemon juice
- ¼ cup Olive oil

Preparation:

1. Put the garlic, basil, oregano, and parsley in a food processor; pulse (for 3 minutes until finely chopped).

2. Form a thick paste by Drizzling the olive oil on the pesto. Scrape down the sides as well. Add the pulse and lemon juice; Blend.

3. Take a sealed container and store the pesto in it; Refrigerate (for one week).

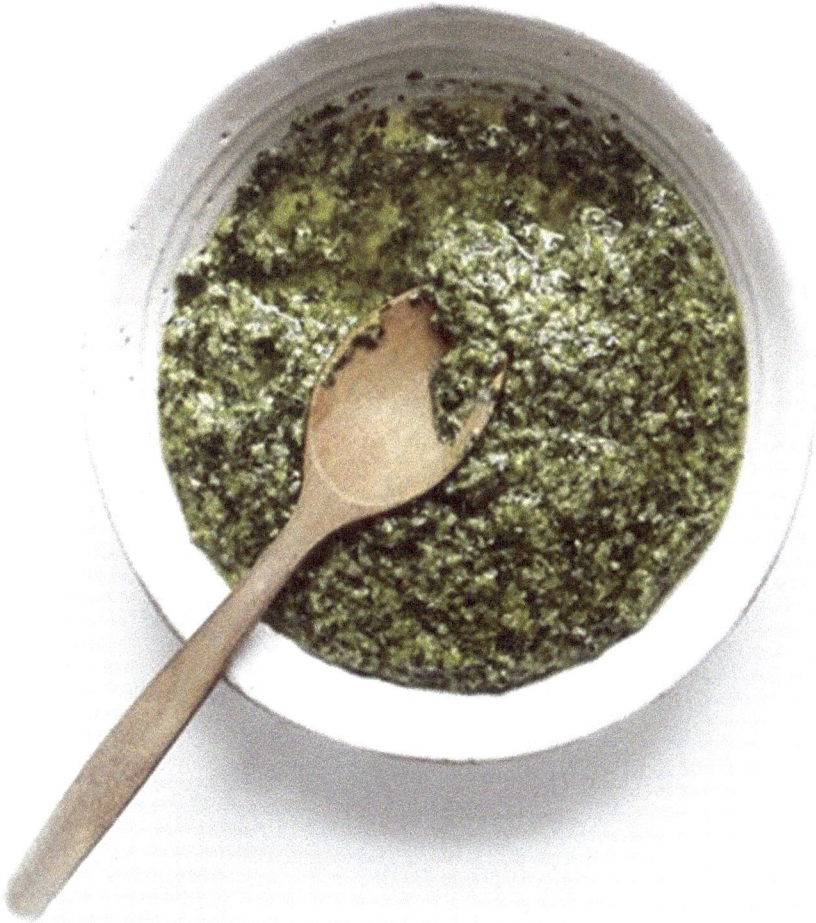

Smoothie Bowl

Prep Time: 4 min

Cook Time: 0 min

Serve: 1

Ingredients:

- 1 tbsp shredded coconut

- ¾ cup blueberries

- 1 tsp Honey

- ½ sliced banana

- 3 tbsp plain coconut milk

- 1 tbsp Blueberries

- ½ cup of Organic and Frozen strawberries

- ½ cup Water

Preparation:

1. Combine all the smoothie bowl ingredients (except coconut and fresh berries) in a high-speed blender.

2. Allow all the ingredients to be like a creamy sorbet; blend.

3. Pour the mixture into a bowl Garnish the smoothie with coconut and fresh berries. Eat!

Irish Colcannon

Prep Time: 5 min

Cook Time: 30 min

Serve: 6

Ingredients:

- 85 g Russet potato

- Three Parsnips

- 1.5 cup Green peas

- 1 cup Green cabbage

- One diced Onion

- 1 cup chopped Kale

- 3 tbsp Olive oil

- Black pepper to taste

- Two minced Garlic cloves

- Sea salt

Preparation:

1. Place potato and parsnips in a pot of water (large) and bring the ingredients to a boil. Cook until tender (over high heat) for about fifteen minutes.

2. Use a sieve to remove the cooked vegetables. Do not drain the remaining cooking liquid left in the pot; reserve for later. Take a shallow bowl, and with 1/3 cup of the cooking liquid and 2 tbsp. Of the olive oil, mash the vegetables in it. 3. Keep adding as much cooking liquid as required to remove the lumps. You can also use a hand blender.

4. Layout mashed parsnip mixture on a foil-covered plate.

5. Now, add chopped kale and shredded cabbage to the parsnip water. Cook until the cabbage is just slack (for a few minutes). For this step, drain the kale and cabbage thoroughly and return them to the pot. Cover.

6. Take a skillet (large) and heat 1 tbsp of olive oil in it using medium heat. Add and cook the chopped garlic and onion until it softens.

7. Further, also add the cooked garlic and onions to the pot with the greens and cabbage. Now also add the peas.

8. In the middle of an empty serving bowl, place the parsnip and potato mash. Add and mix the cooked vegetables in. Season with salt and pepper. Serve! (As lunch or as a side dish).

Vegan Banana Bread

Prep Time: 5 min

Cook Time: 60 min

Serve: 12

Ingredients:

- 1/3 cup Vegetable oil

- 2 tbsp Agave nectar

- 1/8 tsp Salt

- 1.5 cup Whole wheat flour

- ½ cup Applesauce

- 1 tsp Baking soda

- Four Bananas

- 1.5 tsp Vanilla extract

- ½ Sugar

- 4 tbsp Flax seeds

Preparation:

1. Preheat the oven to 350°F. Firstly, peel the bananas and then mash the peeled bananas with a fork. Place the mashed bananas in a mixing bowl.

2. Now, take a wooden spoon and mix the mashed bananas with vegetable oil using it.

3. Add sugar, applesauce, salt, vanilla, baking soda, agave nectar, and ground flaxseeds in the bowl; stir.

4. Add flour and Stir thoroughly. Pour the mixture into a 9 x 5 x 3-inch loaf pan (greased).

5. Bake for a good 50-60 minutes, until the (top) springs back become slightly depressed. Cool and serve!

Vegetable Broth

Prep Time: 10 min

Cook Time: 60 min

Serve: 2

Ingredients:

- 2 cups Sliced celery stalks

- 2 tbsp Olive oil

- Four chopped carrots

- Two chopped onions

- ½ tsp Dried thyme

- Eight cups Water

- ¼ cup Italian parsley

- Two Bay leaves

- 4 Garlic cloves

- 1 tsp Black peppercorns

Preparation:

1. Take a large saucepan, and heat oil in it over medium heat. Add garlic, celery, carrots, and onions. Cook and stir (occasionally) for about 5 minutes.

2. Add peppercorns, water, thyme, parsley, and bay leaves. Set the heat to high now. Bring it to a boil. Now stir again while also reducing heat to medium-low.

3. Let the mixture simmer for about an hour, uncovered.

4. Take a fine-mesh strainer and place it over a large pot. Pour all contents into the strainer. Reserve the broth while discarding the solids.

Festive Cranberry Stuffing

Prep Time: 5 min

Cook Time: 30 min

Serve: 4

Ingredients:

- 1 cup diced tart apples

- ¼ tsp Poultry seasoning

- 3 cups Soft bread

- 2 tbsp butter

- ¼ cup Apple juice

- ¼ cup chopped celery

- ½ cup diced cranberries

Preparation:

1. Preheat the oven to 350°F. Take a large bowl. In it, combine all ingredients; toss and mix.

2. Take a casserole dish (lightly greased). Place the mixture in it and Bake for 30 minutes.

Simple Puerto Rican Sofrito

Prep Time: 5 min

Cook Time: 0 min

Serve: 24

Ingredients:

- One chopped Spanish onion

- 1 tsp salt

- Five Stemmed aji dulce peppers

- One bunch Cilantro

- 1 Chopped green pepper

- 10 Garlic cloves

Preparation:

1. Wash all the ingredients thoroughly before using.

2. Take a blender. Add onions first, and then add all the other ingredients (in small batches).

3. To use within a week, you will be required to refrigerate a portion of your sofrito (in an airtight container. To use within four months or so, freeze in in an ice cube tray or small containers. It is not required to thaw before cooking.

4. Add 2 tbsp. Of sofrito if and whenever you make rice, soups, beans, and stews!

Vegetable Curry

Prep Time: 30 min

Cook Time: 30 min

Serve: 5

Ingredients:

- 1 tsp Fennel seeds

- 1 tsp Cumin seeds

- 1 tbsp Coconut oil

- Two cups Basmati rice

- 1 tsp Coriander seeds

- 1 tsp Mustard seeds

- 1 tsp Hot chili flakes

- ¼ tsp Black peppercorns

- One grated ginger

- One chopped Onion

- 1 tsp Turmeric

- One chopped Carrot

- 6 oz Coconut milk

- 1.5 cups chopped Cauliflower

- One cup Green peas

Preparation:

1. Take a cast-iron skillet, and add dry spices to it. Heat (low-medium heat) for 2 minutes. Cook the rice while the spices are heating up. (As per the DIRECTIONS on the package). Add coconut oil and sauté for about 2-3 minutes (low-medium heat). Heat until the spices start popping and turn brownish.

2. Add ginger, hot chili flakes, and turmeric. Cook (low-medium heat) until aromatic for about six minutes.

3. Remove from heat make a paste of the cooked spices by blending them with the onion.

4. Take a separate pan, and heat the coconut milk in it until it starts to bubble up. Add the spice paste; whisk.

5. Add all the vegetables and for 10 minutes, let them simmer until tender. Serve over rice (as per need).

Tabbouleh

Prep Time: 30 min

Cook Time: 0 min

Serve: 4

Ingredients:

- One cup bulgur

- One cup sliced Cucumbers

- One cup sliced Radish

- Four sliced scallions

- One bunch of Chopped mint leaves

- 2 tbsp lemon juice

- ½ cup olive oil

- Pepper to taste

- Kosher salt to taste

Preparation:

1. Fill a large bowl halfway with hot tap water and stir bulgur into it for 20 to 30 minutes. Let it absorb water enough to not be mushy but soft. In a large bowl, put mint and the vegetables sliced earlier.

2. Drain excess water off the bulgur by squeezing, one at a time. Squeeze tightly by holding it over a sink or a sieve, adding each bulgur squeezed into the vegetable bowl.

3. Add olive oil and lemon juice into the salad. Blend all the ingredients by using either a large spoon or hands. Add salt and pepper with seasoning to taste (if desired). Serve it as a side dish for dinner or with crusty bread as a lunch. Enjoy!

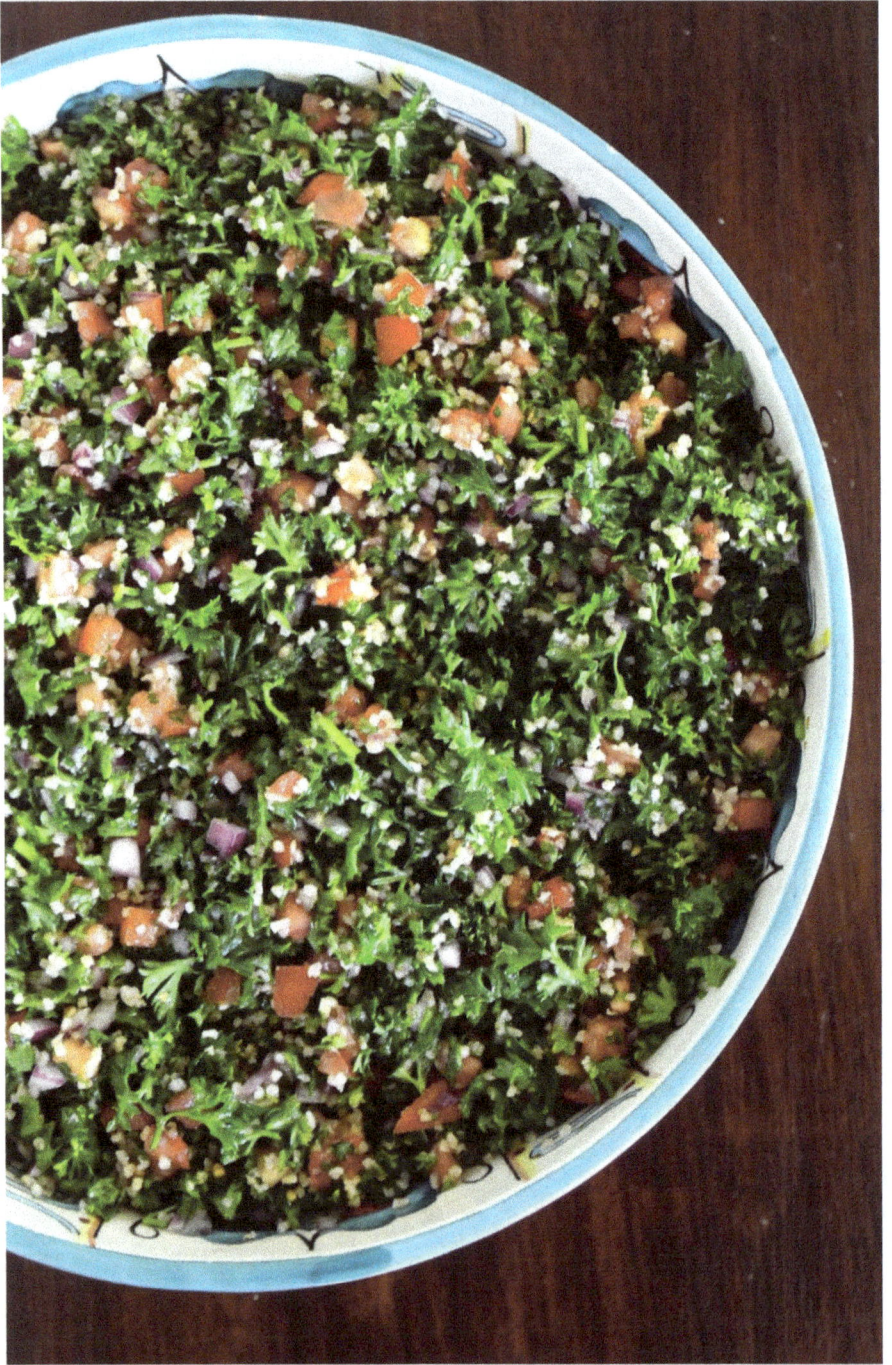

Stuffed Poblano Peppers

Prep Time: 20 min

Cook Time: 30 min

Serve: 5

Ingredients:

- 46 g Poblano peppers

- Two cups of water

- One cup quinoa

- 3 tbsp olive oil

- One diced onion

- Two diced ribs celery

- Two diced carrots

- Two minced garlic cloves

- ½ cup diced red peppers roasted

- 1 tbsp adobo sauce with chipotle

- One cup peas

- 1/3 cup chopped pecans

Preparation:

1. Heat the oven before 375°F. With stem, slit each pepper lengthwise. Scoop the seeds out and put them aside.

2. Take a medium saucepan, heat water, and add quinoa. Until cooked, boil it and simmer with water immersed. Put it aside. Add olive oil in a medium heated skillet.

3. Sauté the carrots, onion, and celery for about 8 minutes until softened. Then add garlic and for a minute sauté it.

4. Add quinoa cooked before in it and mix well. Add the chipotle, pecans, peas, and roasted red peppers.

5. A shallow baking dish places stuffed peppers and bake them until the peppers are softened for 30 minutes.

6. Serve with meat or a side salad. Enjoy!

Shiitake, Soba Noodles, and Miso Bowl

Prep Time: 5 min

Cook Time: 15 min

Serve: 2

Ingredients:

- Three cups of water
- ½ cup dried shiitake mushrooms
- 4 oz soba noodles
- 1 tbsp white miso

Preparation:

1. In a medium saucepan, boil water over high heat. Add mushrooms and cook them for 6 minutes until swollen and softened. Add in the noodles and cook until al dente.

2. Measure one by 4 cups of noodle broth. Add the miso to it and mix thoroughly with a fork or whisk.

3. Pour this mixture back into the saucepan. Serve in bowls.

Collard and Rice Stuffed Red Peppers

Prep Time: 10 min

Cook Time: 50 min

Serve: 4

Ingredients:

- Two red bell peppers
- 2 tbsp olive oil
- Black pepper to taste
- Six cups collard greens
- ½ chopped sweet onion
- Three minced garlic cloves
- One cup of white rice cooked
- 2 tbsp lemon Juice
- ¼ cup roasted sunflower seeds

Preparation:

1. Preheat oven at 400°F. Cut half the peppers and remove the stems and seeds. Brush the inside and out with one tbsp of olive oil. Spice them with pepper and put the baking dish cut side down.

2. Until just tender, bake them for ten to fifteen minutes. Flip-up the cut- side of peppers after removing them from the oven and leave the oven on.

3. Take a large saucepan and boil four cups of water. Cook collard greens in it until just tender, for about five to seven minutes. Drain and rinse them under cold water. Then Chop them finely. Take a large skillet, and at medium heat, put the left behind tbsp of olive oil. Add in the onion, stir and cook for five to seven minutes, until it turns brown. Add in and cook garlic until it is fragrant.

4. Mix in the collard greens. Put it off from the stove, and add rice and lemon juice in it. Spice it up with pepper.

5. Divide this filling into the pepper halves and crest each half with one tbsp of sunflower seeds. Add one by the fourth cup of water in a baking dish, wrap it with aluminum foil. Bake it for twenty minutes, until it is heated through. Uncover it and then bake again for five more minutes.

Ginger yogurt dresses the citrus salad

Prep Time: 15 min

Cook Time: 0 min

Serve: 6

Ingredients:

- One grapefruit

- Two tangerines

- 2/3 cup ginger

- 1/4 cup sugar

- 2 tbsp honey

- Three navel oranges

- 1/2 cup cranberries

- 1/4 tsp cinnamon

- 17.6 oz Greek yogurt

Preparation:

1. Break the grapefruit. Cut grapefruit threads, cut the tangerine sections into half. Transfer the grapefruit, all juices & tangerines into a deep serving bowl.

2. Use a small sharp knife, Slice oranges into round shapes and slices into quarters. Add oranges & all juices into a bowl. Mix in cranberries, cinnamon & honey.

3. Cover & refrigerate for 1 hour. Then Mix yogurt & ginger in a bowl. Sprinkle brown sugar & cranberries.

Grilled halloumi cheese salad

Prep Time: 10 min

Cook Time: 5 min

Serve: 4

Ingredients:

- Salad

- 8 oz Halloumi cheese

- 1 cup black olives

- 1/2 cup green olives

- 2 cups tomatoes

- 4 cups arugula

- 1 tbsp olive oil

- 4 cups shishito peppers

- 1 cup mint leaves

- 1/2 cup chives

- Honey Citrus Dressing

- One garlic cloves

- 1 tsp Dijon mustard

- 2 tsp honey

- 2 tsp lemon juice

- 1/4 cup olive oil salt and pepper

- 1 tsp thyme optional

- Chili optional

Preparation:

1. Cut down the cheese into 0.5-inch slices and soak them in water if required. Heat the grill pan & then adds olive oil to it. Take the cheese slices and grill every slice for 1 to 2 minutes, from one side. Remove the cheese, add the peppers, & increase the temp.

2. Let the peppers cook for three minutes per side. Let the peppers cool down & then chop them with the cheese into small cubes. Mix these with the remaining salad items.

3. Transfer everything in a small bowl and Enjoy.

Herbed calamari salad

Prep Time: 20 min

Cook Time: 5 min

Serve: 6

Ingredients:

- 3 tbsp extra virgin olive oil

- Two minced garlic cloves

- 2.5 lb calamari rings

- 1/4 cup cilantro leaves

- 1/2 cup leaf parsley leaves

- 3/4 tsp kosher salt

- 1/4 tsp black pepper

- One pinch of red pepper

- juice of one lemon

- 1/4 cup mint leaves

- Sliced peel of one lemon

Preparation:

1. Defrost the calamari. With the help of a cutting, the knife removes skin from the preserved lemon. Remove the inside portion & Slice them into thin pieces.

2. Chop garlic & mince also chop washed parsley, cilantro, & mint. Heat frying pan at high temperature and the add 1.5tbsp. of olive oil to it. Heat oil again and add garlic to it and cook with continuous stirring for 20-30 sec. Cook until it is scented, then add calamari batches in it. Divide the 1.5 tbsp. Olive oil in it and cook the calamari batches.

3. Add a pinch of Black pepper & sea salt & continue cooking for 2 to 4 minutes. Or cook until it becomes opaque & firm. Do not overcook it otherwise, it becomes a rubber-like mixture. Remove the excess liquid left during cooking and convert the coked calamari into a mixing bowl.

4. Add remaining pepper, olive oil, salt, red pepper, preserved lemon rind, herbs, & lemon juice in a mixing bowl & cook well while calamari still warm.

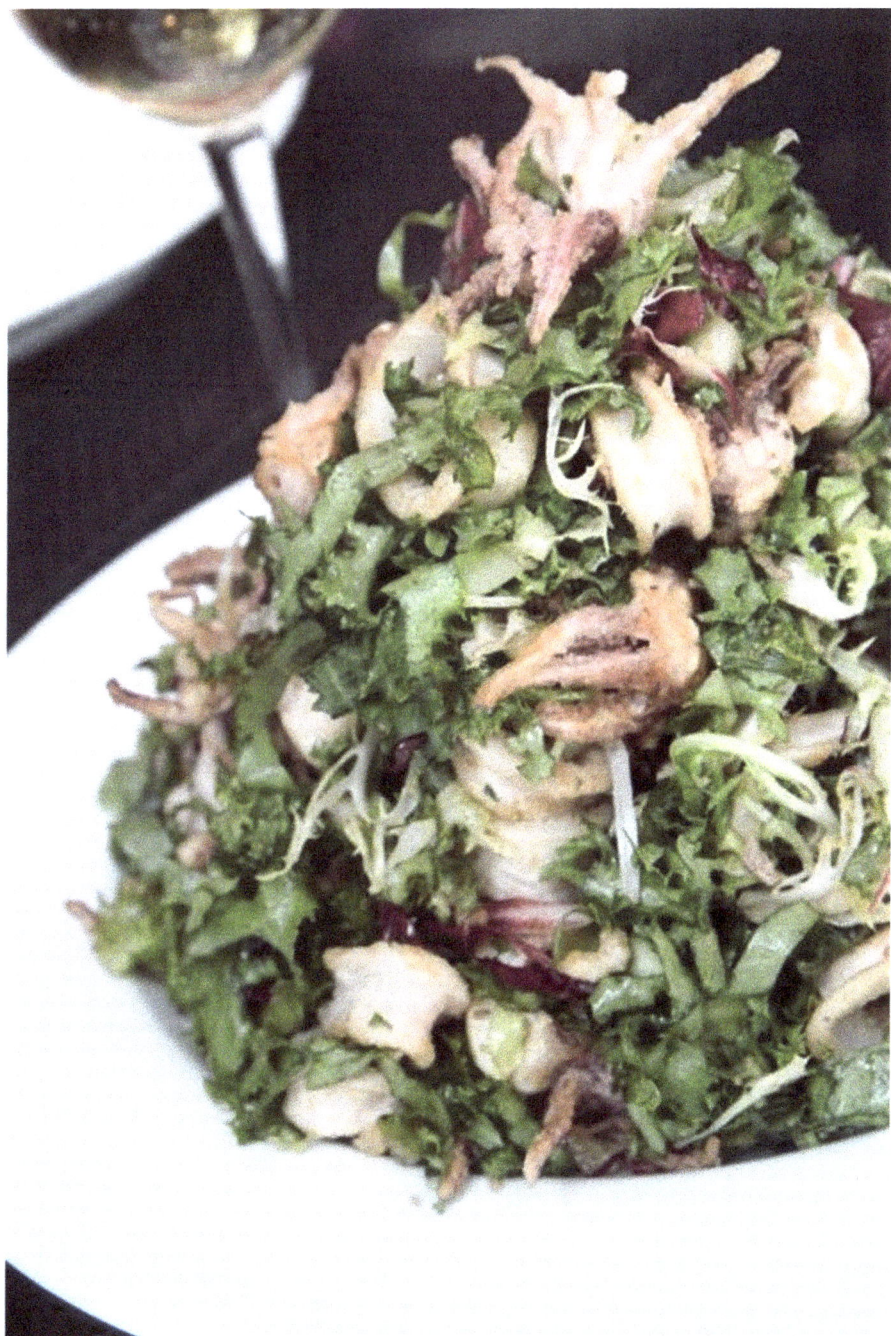

www.ingramcontent.com/pod-product-compliance
Lightning Source LLC
Chambersburg PA
CBHW050746030426
42336CB00012B/1684